Elder Women's Diabetic Delights

Flavourful Recipes for Blood Sugar Management

By Dr. Marcia Moss

Copyright ©2023 by Dr. Marcia Moss.

Table of Content

INTRODUCTION: 5

SUSTAINABLE DIABETIS GUIDE HEALTH AND WELL-BEING 8

UNDERSTANDING DIABETES AND AGING 8

BONE HEALTH AND DIABETES 9

MEDICATION MANAGEMENT AND BLOOD 10

SUGAR CONTROL 10

BALANCED NUTRITION FOR ELDER WOMEN WITH DIABETES 10

FLAVORFUL RECIPES FOR BLOOD SUGAR 11

MANAGEMENT 11

PRACTICAL TIPS FOR EVERYDAY LIVING 12

MONITORING AND PROGRESS 13

RECIPES FOR BLOOD SUGAR 14

MANAGEMENT 14

BREAKFAST OPTIONS: 14

1. Greek Yogurt Parfait 14

   - Ingredients: 14

   - Instructions: 14

2. Oatmeal with Almonds and Cinnamon 15

   - Ingredients: 15

   - Instructions: 15

3. Veggie Omelette 16

   - Ingredients: 16

LUNCH AND DINNER IDEAS 18

4. Grilled Chicken Salad 18

   - Ingredients: 18

   - Instructions: 18

5. Baked Salmon with Steamed Broccoli and Quinoa 19

   - Ingredients: 19

   - Instructions: 19

6. Lentil Soup 20

   - Ingredients: 20

- Instructions: 20

SNACK OPTIONS: 22

7. Apple Slices with Peanut Butter 22
- Ingredients: 22
8. Veggie Sticks with Hummus 23
- Ingredients: 23

FLAVORFUL DINNERS: 24

9. Stir-Fried Tofu and Vegetables 24
- Ingredients: 24
- Instructions: 24
10. Zucchini Noodles with Pesto 25
- Ingredients: 25
11. Turkey and Vegetable Stir- Fry 26
- Ingredients: 26
- Instructions: 26

DELICIOUS DESSERTS: 27

12. Berry and Yogurt Parfait 27
- Ingredients: 27
13. Dark Chocolate-Dipped Strawberries 28
- Ingredients: 28
14. Chia Seed Pudding 29
- Ingredients: 29
- Instructions: 29

PRACTICAL MEAL PREP: 30

15. Quinoa Salad with Chickpeas and Veggies 30
- Ingredients: 30
- Instructions: 30
16. Roasted Vegetable Medley 31
- Ingredients: 31
- Instructions: 31
17. Overnight Oats with Berries 32
- Ingredients: 32
- Instructions: 32

FLAVORFUL SEASONINGS: 33

18. Herb-Roasted Chicken 33
- Ingredients: 33
- Instructions: 33

19. Lemon-Garlic Shrimp 34
  - Ingredients: 34
  - Instructions: 34
20. Cumin-Spiced Roasted Cauliflower 35
  - Ingredients: 35
  - Instructions: 35
BALANCED LUNCHES: 36
21. Tuna Salad Lettuce Wraps 36
  - Ingredients: 36
  - Instructions: 36
22. Quinoa and Black Bean Bowl 37
  - Ingredients: 37
  - Instructions: 37
23. Spinach and Feta Stuffed Bell Peppers 38
  - Ingredients: 38
SATISFYING SNACKS: 39
24. Cottage Cheese and Berries - Ingredients: 39
  - Instructions: 39
25. Trail Mix 39
  - Ingredients: 39
  - Instructions: 40
26. Rice Cake with Hummus and Cucumber 40
  - Ingredients: 40
  - Instructions: 40
EASY DINNERS: 41
27. Baked Chicken and Sweet Potatoes 41
  - Ingredients: 41
  - Instructions: 41
28. Lentil and Vegetable Stir- Fry 42
  - Ingredients: 42
  - Instructions: 42
39. Baked Salmon with Lemon-Dill Sauce 43
  - Ingredients: 43
  - Instructions: 43

CONCLUSION: 44

THANKS FOR READING: 46

Introduction:

In a world that often races ahead at breakneck speed, it's easy to overlook the quiet strength and wisdom that comes with age. Life's journey has granted our elders a treasury of experience, and when it comes to health, few things are as important as managing blood sugar levels.

Welcome to a culinary adventure that celebrates the resilience and vitality of elder women while unlocking the secrets to a delicious and balanced diabetic-friendly diet.

In the heartwarming pages of "Elder Women's Diabetic Delights: Flavorful Recipes for Blood Sugar Management," we invite you to join us on a journey that combines the wisdom of our seasoned cooks with the innovative techniques of modern nutritional science.

This isn't just another cookbook; it's a tribute to the joy of cooking, the art of eating well, and the undeniable strength of the human spirit.

Allow us to introduce you to Jennifer, a remarkable woman whose story encapsulates the essence of this book. At the age of 68, Jennifer found herself at a crossroads. A diagnosis of type 2 diabetes had seemingly halted her zest for life. Yet, in the midst of uncertainty, she discovered an unwavering determination to regain control of her health.

Armed with a desire to savor life's flavors while managing her blood sugar, Jennifer embarked on a culinary exploration that led her to the heart of this book.

Jennifer's journey, a relatable testament to the challenges many elder women face, resonates deeply within these pages. As we share her experiences, struggles, and triumphs, we'll guide you through a treasure trove of recipes specifically designed to harmonize with a diabetic lifestyle.

We firmly believe that food should not only nourish the body but also enliven the soul, and this book is a testament to that belief.

Our approach is simple: we've brought together a collection of easy-to-follow recipes that celebrate the natural flavors of wholesome ingredients. These dishes are tailored to ensure that they don't just maintain stable blood sugar levels but delight the taste buds and inspire the chef within you.

From hearty breakfasts that greet each day with a smile to satisfying dinners that bring families together around the table, each recipe is a step towards a healthier, happier you.

"Elder Women's Diabetic Delights" is more than just a cookbook; it's an invitation to a brighter, more flavorful future.

Let these pages be your guide as you embark on a culinary journey that honors the wisdom of age, embraces the joy of food, and empowers you to take charge of your health.

With Jennifer's story as a beacon of hope, and these recipes as your compass, we invite you to step into a world where delicious possibilities and balanced well-being converge.

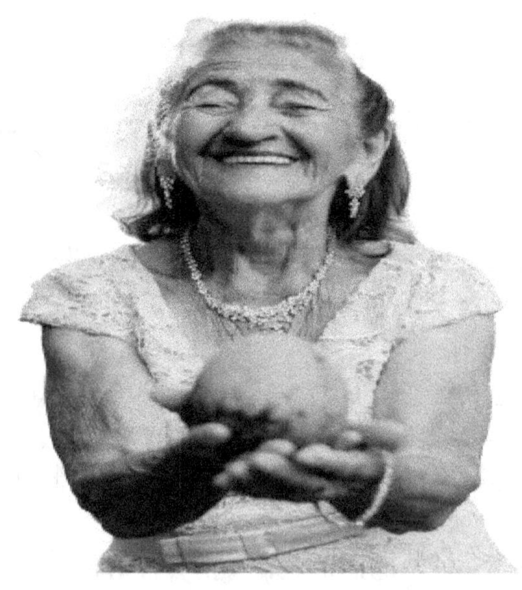

Sustainable Diabetes Guide to Health and Well-Being

Understanding Diabetes and Aging

Diabetes, a chronic metabolic disorder, affects a substantial portion of elder women, with its prevalence rising as people age.

This can be attributed to factors such as decreased insulin sensitivity and impaired glucose regulation. Managing diabetes becomes increasingly challenging with age due to various physiological changes that affect blood sugar control.

The decline in muscle mass and physical activity can lead to insulin resistance, while hormonal shifts may impact insulin production and utilization. Therefore, tailoring diabetes management strategies to individual needs becomes crucial.

One significant approach is personalized dietary intervention. Elder women with diabetes can benefit from customized meal plans that consider their specific nutritional requirements, preferences, and lifestyle.

These diets should prioritize complex carbohydrates with a low glycemic index, promoting gradual blood sugar elevation. Adequate fiber intake assists in stabilizing glucose levels and managing weight, reducing the risk of cardiovascular complications often associated with diabetes.

Bone Health and Diabetes

Diabetes and aging can synergistically impact bone health. Research suggests a connection between diabetes and decreased bone density, potentially increasing the risk of fractures and osteoporosis.

Balancing blood sugar levels is vital for preventing bone loss, as chronic hyperglycemia can impair bone-forming cells and disrupt the bone remodeling process.

To support bone health, elder women with diabetes should adopt dietary strategies rich in bone-strengthening nutrients. Calcium and vitamin D are pivotal for maintaining bone density, and foods like dairy products, leafy greens, and fatty fish can provide these nutrients.

Additionally, foods containing magnesium, phosphorus, and vitamin K contribute to overall bone integrity.

Medication Management and Blood Sugar Control

Effective diabetes management often involves medication, particularly as people age and insulin production wanes. It's essential for elder women to understand the medications they are prescribed, including their mechanisms of action, potential side effects, and interactions with other drugs. Proper medication management involves adhering to prescribed dosages and timings, and being aware of how these factors may change with age.

Nutrition plays a complementary role in medication effectiveness. Consistent blood sugar control can be achieved by aligning meal composition and timing with medication schedules. Moreover, certain nutrients, like chromium and magnesium, are associated with improved insulin sensitivity and glucose metabolism.

Balanced Nutrition for Elder Women with Diabetes

Macronutrients play a critical role in managing blood sugar levels for elder women with diabetes. Carbohydrates should be chosen wisely, focusing on whole grains, vegetables, and legumes, while limiting refined sugars and processed foods. Proteins help stabilize blood sugar levels and promote satiety, making lean sources like poultry, fish, tofu, and legumes valuable choices. Healthy fats, such as those found in avocados, nuts, and olive oil, aid in nutrient absorption and support heart health.

Portion control is essential to prevent overeating and maintain steady glucose levels. Awareness of hunger and fullness cues can be improved by using mindful eating practices like eating deliberately and savoring each bite.. Crafting balanced meals involves incorporating a variety of nutrient-rich foods to ensure a well-rounded diet.

Flavorful Recipes for Blood Sugar Management

Elder women with diabetes can enjoy a diverse range of flavorful and nutritious meals. For breakfast, options like Greek yogurt with berries and nuts provide protein and fiber without causing rapid blood sugar spikes. Lunch and dinner ideas include grilled chicken salads with colorful vegetables and quinoa, showcasing a balance of macronutrients.

Snacks can consist of carrot sticks with hummus or a handful of mixed nuts, contributing to sustained energy levels throughout the day.

Culinary creativity can enhance the dining experience without compromising health goals. Utilizing herbs, spices, and citrus flavors can elevate dishes while minimizing the need for excessive salt or added sugars.

Practical Tips for Everyday Living

Staying physically active is key to managing diabetes and promoting overall well-being in elder women. Engaging in regular exercise routines tailored to individual abilities and preferences can help maintain muscle mass, improve insulin sensitivity, and enhance cardiovascular health. Activities like walking, swimming, and gentle yoga can be effective options.

Coping with stress is equally important, as it can impact blood sugar levels. Elder women should explore relaxation techniques such as deep breathing, meditation, or engaging in hobbies to manage stress effectively.

Navigating social situations and dining out may require planning and communication, ensuring that dietary needs are met without sacrificing enjoyment or social interaction.

Special occasions can be enjoyed mindfully by focusing on portion sizes and making conscious food choices.

Monitoring and Progress

The main cornerstone of diabetes management is regular blood sugar monitoring. Elder women should understand their target ranges and how different foods, activities, and medications can influence glucose readings. Tracking progress allows for adjustments to be made to the dietary and lifestyle plan as needed. Consulting healthcare professionals regularly provides valuable insights and guidance on optimizing diabetes management.

In General, managing diabetes in elder women requires a comprehensive approach that considers the interplay of aging, medication management, nutrition, and emotional well-being. Tailored strategies, along with the support of healthcare professionals, empower these women to lead fulfilling lives while effectively managing their diabetes.

Recipes for Blood Sugar Management

Breakfast Options:

1. Greek Yogurt Parfait

- Ingredients:

- 1 cup Greek yogurt
- half cup mixed berries (Rasberries, blueberries, strawberries, etc)
- 2 tablespoons of chopped nuts (almonds, walnuts, etc)

- Instructions:

1. In a glass or bowl, layer Greek yogurt, mixed berries, and chopped nuts.
2. Repeat the layers until the ingredients are used up.
3. Enjoy immediately or let it refrigerate for later.

2. Oatmeal with Almonds and Cinnamon

- Ingredients:

- 1/2 cup rolled oats
- 1 cup almond milk (unsweetened)
- 1 tablespoon chopped almonds
- 1/2 teaspoon cinnamon
- 1 teaspoon honey or maple syrup (optional)

- Instructions:

1. In a saucepan, bring almond milk to a gentle boil.
2. Stir in rolled oats and reduce heat to a simmer. Cook for 5-7 minutes, stirring occasionally.
3. Once the oatmeal reaches your desired consistency, remove from heat.
4. Transfer oatmeal to a bowl and top with chopped almonds, cinnamon, and sweetener if desired.

3. Veggie Omelette

- Ingredients:

- 2 eggs
- 1/2 cup chopped spinach
- 1/4 cup diced bell peppers
- 2 tablespoons crumbled feta cheese
- Salt and pepper to taste - Cooking spray or olive oil

- Instructions:

1. In a bowl, whisk the eggs thoroughly until well beaten. Season with salt and pepper.

2. Heat a non-stick skillet over medium heat and coat with cooking spray or a small amount of olive oil.

3. Add the chopped spinach and bell peppers to the skillet and sauté for about 2 minutes until slightly softened.

4. Pour the whisked eggs over the vegetables. Allow the eggs to cook for a minute or so, undisturbed.

5. Once the edges are set, gently lift the edges of the omelette with a spatula and tilt the skillet to let the uncooked egg flow to the edges.

6. Sprinkle crumbled feta cheese over one half of the omelette.

7. Carefully fold the other half of the omelette over the cheese.

8. Cook for another minute or until the eggs are fully set and the cheese is melted.

9. Slide the omelette onto a plate and serve.

Lunch and Dinner Ideas

4. Grilled Chicken Salad

- Ingredients:

- 4 oz grilled chicken breast
- 2 cups mixed salad greens (lettuce, arugula, spinach)
- 1/4 cup cherry tomatoes, halved
- 1/4 cup cucumber slices
- 2 tablespoons balsamic vinaigrette dressing

- Instructions:

1. Season the chicken breast with your choice of seasonings (salt, pepper, herbs).

2. Over medium-high heat, Preheat a grill or grill pan.

3. Grill the chicken for about 5-6 minutes on each side, or until cooked through.

4. In a large bowl, combine the salad greens, cherry tomatoes, and cucumber slices.

5. Slice the grilled chicken and place it on top of the salad.

6. Blend the salad by adding the balsamic vinaigrette dressing and tossing.

5. Baked Salmon with Steamed Broccoli and Quinoa

- Ingredients:

- 4 oz salmon fillet
- 1/2 cup cooked quinoa
- 1 cup steamed broccoli florets
- Lemon wedges
- Olive oil
- Salt and pepper to taste

- Instructions:

1. Set the oven to 375°F (190°C) before using it.
2. On a baking sheet with parchment paper, arrange the salmon fillet.
3. Drizzle the salmon with a little olive oil and season with salt and pepper.
4. The salmon should bake for 12 to 15 minutes in the preheated oven, or until it flakes easily with a fork.
5. While the salmon is baking, cook the quinoa according to package instructions.
6. Steam the broccoli florets until tender, about 4-5 minutes.
7. Serve the baked salmon on a plate alongside the cooked quinoa and steamed broccoli.
8. Squeeze fresh lemon juice over the salmon before enjoying.

6. Lentil Soup

- Ingredients:

- 1 cup of rinsed and drained dried green or brown lentils,
    - 1 onion, chopped
    - 2 carrots, peeled and chopped
    - 2 celery stalks, chopped
    - 2 cloves garlic, minced
    - 6 cups of chicken broth or low-sodium vegetable
    - 1 teaspoon ground cumin
    - 1/2 teaspoon ground turmeric
    - Salt and pepper to taste - Fresh lemon juice (optional
)

- Instructions:

1. In a large pot, sauté the chopped onion, carrots, and celery in a little olive oil until softened.

2. Add the minced garlic, ground cumin, and ground turmeric to the pot. Allow it to cook for about 1 minute until fragrant.

3. Add the rinsed lentils and broth to the pot. Bring to a boil, then reduce the heat and let simmer for about 25-30 minutes, or until the lentils are tender.

4. Use an immersion blender to partially blend the soup, leaving some lentils whole for texture.

5. Season the soup with salt and pepper to taste.

6. Squeeze a little fresh lemon juice into each serving before enjoying.

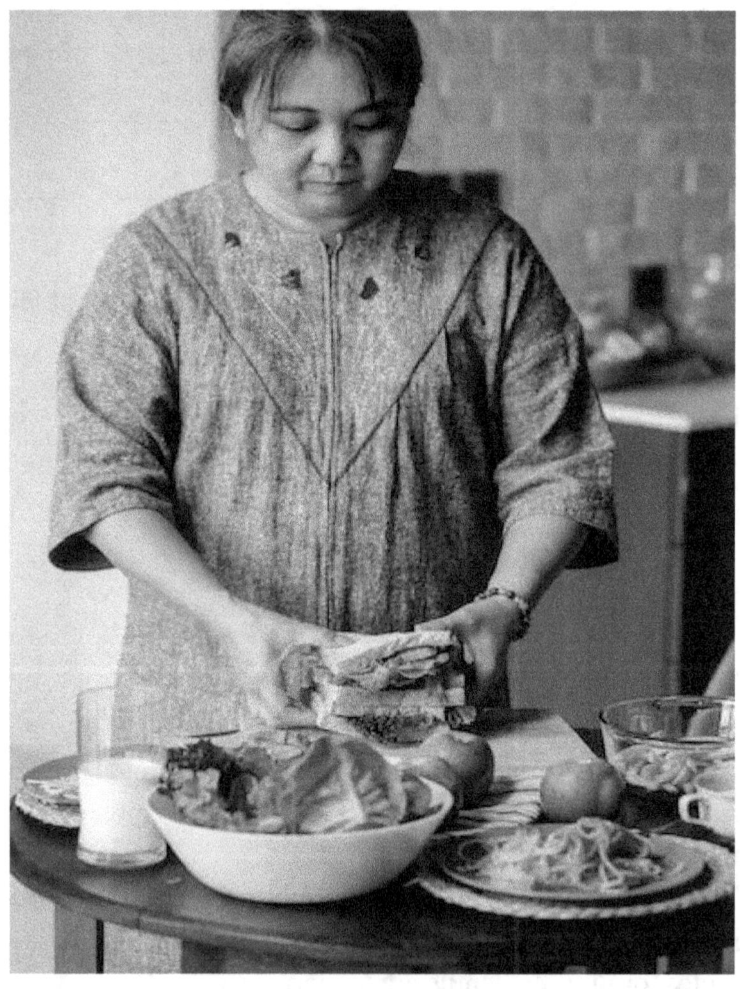

7. Apple Slices with Peanut Butter

- Ingredients:

- 1 medium apple, sliced
- 2 tablespoons natural peanut butter

- Instructions:

1. Slice the apple into thin wedges.
2. Dip each apple slice into the peanut butter before eating.

8. Veggie Sticks with Hummus

- Ingredients:

- Assorted vegetable sticks (carrots, cucumber, bell peppers)

- 1/4 cup hummus

- Instructions:

1. Wash and cut the vegetables into sticks.

2. Serve the vegetable sticks with a side of hummus for dipping.

Flavorful Dinners:

9. Stir-Fried Tofu and Vegetables

- Ingredients:

- 1 cup firm tofu, cubed
- 1 cup mixed vegetables (carrots, bell peppers, broccoli)
- 2 tablespoons low-sodium soy sauce
- 1 teaspoon minced fresh ginger
- 1 garlic clove, minced
- 1 tablespoon sesame oil

- Instructions:

1. Over medium-high heat, Heat sesame oil in a pan.
2. Add minced ginger and garlic, and sauté for about 1 minute.
3. Add cubed tofu and mixed vegetables to the pan. Stir-fry for 5-7 minutes until tofu is lightly browned and vegetables are tender.
4. Drizzle soy sauce over the tofu and vegetables, tossing to coat.
5. Serve over cooked brown rice or quinoa.

10. Zucchini Noodles with Pesto

- Ingredients:

- 2 medium zucchinis, spiralized into noodles
- 1/4 cup homemade or store-bought pesto sauce
- Grated Parmesan cheese (optional)

- Instructions:

1. In a large pan, sauté zucchini noodles over medium heat for 2-3 minutes until slightly softened.

2. Toss the zucchini noodles with pesto sauce until well coated.

3. Serve in a bowl, garnished with grated Parmesan cheese if desired.

11. Turkey and Vegetable Stir- Fry

- Ingredients:

- 1/2 lb lean ground turkey
- 1 cup mixed vegetables (snap peas, bell peppers, carrots)
- 2 tablespoons low-sodium soy sauce
- 1 tablespoon hoisin sauce
- 1 teaspoon sesame oil
- 1 teaspoon minced garlic
- Cooked brown rice for serving

- Instructions:

1. In a skillet, heat sesame oil over medium-high heat.

2. Add minced garlic and ground turkey. Cook cooked through until turkey is browned.

3. Add mixed vegetables to the skillet and stir-fry for 3-4 minutes until vegetables are tender- crisp.

4. Pour soy sauce and hoisin sauce over the turkey and vegetables, tossing to combine.

Delicious Desserts:

When you first find that an elderly family member has diabetes, you might assume that they must permanently exclude desserts from their diet. However, that is simply untrue. Desserts can be enjoyed in moderation by those with diabetes while still maintaining stable blood sugar levels. Making wise dessert choices can also make a difference because not all sweets are made equally. The following dessert suggestions are healthier for diabetics:

12. Berry and Yogurt Parfait

- Ingredients:

- 1 cup low-fat Greek yogurt
- 1/2 cup mixed with berries (blueberries, strawberries, raspberries)
- 2 tablespoons of chopped nuts (walnuts, Almonds) –

Instructions:

1. In a glass or bowl, layer Greek yogurt, mixed berries, and chopped nuts.
2. Repeat the layers until the ingredients are used up.
3. Enjoy immediately.

13. Dark Chocolate-Dipped Strawberries

- Ingredients:

- Fresh strawberries, washed and dried - Dark chocolate (70% cocoa or higher), melted

- Instructions:

1. Melt the dark chocolate using a double boiler or microwave, stirring until smooth.
2. Dip each strawberry into the melted chocolate, allowing excess chocolate to drip off.
3. Place dipped strawberries on a parchment-lined tray and refrigerate until the chocolate sets.

14. Chia Seed Pudding

- Ingredients:

- 2 tablespoons chia seeds
- 1/2 cup unsweetened almond milk
- 1/4 teaspoon vanilla extract - Mixed fresh fruit for topping

- Instructions:

1. In a jar or bowl, combine chia seeds, almond milk, and vanilla extract.

2. Stir well and refrigerate for at least 2 hours or overnight, stirring occasionally.

3. Top the chia pudding with mixed fresh fruit before serving.

Practical Meal Prep:

15. Quinoa Salad with Chickpeas and Veggies

- Ingredients:

- 1 cup cooked quinoa
- 1/2 cup drained and rinsed canned chickpeas,
- 1/2 cup diced cucumber
- 1/4 cup diced red bell pepper
- 2 tablespoons chopped fresh parsley
- Juice of 1 lemon
- 2 tablespoons extra-virgin olive oil
- Salt and pepper to taste

- Instructions:

1. In a large bowl, combine cooked quinoa, chickpeas, cucumber, red bell pepper, and chopped parsley.
2. Drizzle lemon juice and olive oil over the salad, and season with salt and pepper.
3. Toss to combine all ingredients thoroughly.
4. Divide the salad into individual meal prep containers for convenient lunches.

16. Roasted Vegetable Medley

- Ingredients:

- Assorted vegetables (bell peppers, zucchini, carrots, onions)
- Olive oil
- dried herbs, Salt and pepper(such as rosemary or thyme)

- Instructions:

1. Preheat the oven temperature to 400°F (200 °C).

2. Wash, peel, and chop the vegetables into bite-sized pieces.

3. Toss the vegetables with olive oil, salt, pepper, and dried herbs in a mixing bowl.

4. Spread the whole vegetables in a single layer on a baking sheet.

5. Roast in the preheated oven for 20-25 minutes, or until the vegetables are tender and slightly caramelized.

6. Let it cool slightly before dividing into meal prep containers.

17. Overnight Oats with Berries

- Ingredients:

- 1/2 cup rolled oats
- 1/2 cup unsweetened almond milk
- 1/4 cup mixed berries (strawberries, blueberries, Raspberries)
- 1 tablespoon chia seeds
- 1 teaspoon of honey or maple syrup (this is optional)

- Instructions:

1. In a jar or container, combine rolled oats, almond milk, mixed berries, chia seeds, and sweetener if using.
2. Stir well, ensuring all ingredients are combined.
3. Seal the container and refrigerate overnight.
4. In the morning, give the oats a good stir and enjoy cold or gently heated.

18. Herb-Roasted Chicken

- Ingredients:

- 2 boneless, skinless chicken breasts
- 2 tablespoons olive oil
- 1 teaspoon of dried mixed herbs (such as rosemary, thyme or rosemary)
- Salt and pepper to taste

- Instructions:

1. Preheat the oven temperature to 375°F (190 °C).
2. Rub the chicken breasts with olive oil, dried herbs, salt, and pepper.
3. Place the seasoned chicken on a baking sheet.
4. Roast in the preheated oven for 25-30 minutes or until the chicken is cooked through and juices run clear.
5. Let the chicken rest for a few minutes before slicing.

19. Lemon-Garlic Shrimp

- Ingredients:

- 1/2 lb of peeled and deveined large shrimp
- Zest and juice of 1 lemon
- 2 cloves garlic, minced
- 1 tablespoon olive oil
- Salt and pepper to taste

- Instructions:

1.   Combine the lemon zest, lemon juice, garlic powder, olive oil, salt, and pepper in a bowl.

2.   Include the shrimp in the bowl, peeling and deveining them first.

3.   Turn up the heat on a skillet to medium-high.

4.   Add the marinated shrimp to the skillet and cook for 2-3 minutes per side until pink and cooked through.

5.   Serve the shrimp with your choice of sides.

20. Cumin-Spiced Roasted Cauliflower

- Ingredients:

- 1 head cauliflower, cut into florets
- 2 tablespoons olive oil
- 1 teaspoon ground cumin
- Salt and pepper to taste

- Instructions:

1. Preheat the oven temperature to 400°F (200 °C).
2. In a large bowl, toss cauliflower florets with olive oil, ground cumin, salt, and pepper.
3. Arrange the cauliflower in a single layer on a baking pan.
4. Roast the cauliflower for 20 to 25 minutes, or until it is soft and golden brown, in the preheated oven.
5. Serve the roasted cauliflower as a flavorful side dish.

21. Tuna Salad Lettuce Wraps

- Ingredients:

- 1 can of tuna in water, drained.
- 2 tablespoons Greek yogurt or mayonnaise
- 1 celery stalk, finely chopped
- 1 tablespoon chopped red onion - Salt and pepper to taste
- Large lettuce leaves (such as Romaine or butter lettuce)

- Instructions:

1. In a bowl, mix together drained tuna, Greek yogurt (or mayonnaise), chopped celery, small chopped red onion, salt, and pepper.
2. Spoon the tuna salad onto large lettuce leaves and wrap to make lettuce wraps.
3. Secure with toothpicks if needed and enjoy.

22. Quinoa and Black Bean Bowl

- Ingredients:

- 1 cup cooked quinoa
- ½ of drained and rinsed cup canned black beans,
- 1/4 cup diced bell peppers
- 1/4 cup diced avocado
- 2 tablespoons chopped cilantro
- Juice of 1 lime
- Salt and pepper to taste

- Instructions:

1. In a bowl, combine cooked quinoa, black beans, diced bell peppers, diced avocado, chopped cilantro, lime juice, salt, and pepper.

2. Toss to combine all ingredients.

3. Serve as a nutritious and flavorful bowl.

23. Spinach and Feta Stuffed Bell Peppers

- Ingredients:

- 2 bell peppers, halved and seeds removed
- 1 cup cooked quinoa
- 1 cup chopped spinach
- 1/4 cup crumbled feta cheese
- 1/4 cup diced tomatoes
- 1 teaspoon olive oil - Salt and pepper to taste

-Instructions:

1. Preheat the oven temperature to 375°F (190°C).
2. heat olive oil over medium heat in a skillet.
3. Add well chopped spinach and cook until properly wilted.
4. In a bowl, mix together cooked quinoa, wilted spinach, crumbled feta cheese, diced tomatoes, salt, and pepper.
5. 5.In the quinoa mixture,
6. Stuff the bell pepper halves.
7. Place the stuffed peppers on a baking sheet and bake in the preheated oven for 20-25 minutes, or until the peppers are tender.

Satisfying Snacks:

24. Cottage Cheese and Berries

- Ingredients:

- 1/2 cup low-fat cottage cheese
- 1/4 cup mixed berries (strawberries, blueberries, raspberries)

- Instructions:

1. In a bowl, top the cottage cheese with mixed berries.
2. Enjoy as a protein-packed snack.

25. Trail Mix

- Ingredients:

- Mixed nuts (almonds, walnuts, cashews)
- Dried fruit (raisins, dried cranberries)
- Dark chocolate chips (optional)

- Instructions:

1. Mix together nuts, dried fruit, and dark chocolate chips in a bowl.
2. Portion the trail mix into individual snack-sized bags for convenient on-the-go snacking.

26. Rice Cake with Hummus and Cucumber

- Ingredients:

- Plain rice cake
- 2 tablespoons hummus
- Sliced cucumber

- Instructions:

1. Spread hummus thoroughly on a rice cake.
2. Top with sliced cucumber.
3. Enjoy as a light and crunchy snack.

27. Baked Chicken and Sweet Potatoes

- Ingredients:

- 2 boneless, skinless chicken breasts
- 1 medium sweet potato, diced and   peeled
- 1 tablespoon olive oil
- 1 teaspoon dried rosemary
- Salt and pepper to taste

- Instructions:

1. Preheat the oven temperature to 400°F (200 °C).

2. Place chicken breasts on one side of a baking sheet.

3. Toss diced sweet potatoes with olive oil, dried rosemary, salt, and pepper. Spread them on the other side of the baking sheet.

4. Bake in the preheated oven for 20-25 minutes, or until the chicken is cooked through and the sweet potatoes are tender.

28. Lentil and Vegetable Stir- Fry

- Ingredients:

- 1 cup cooked brown or green lentils
- 1 cup mixed vegetables (carrots, bell peppers, broccoli)
- 2 tablespoons low-sodium soy sauce
- 1 tablespoon hoisin sauce
- 1 teaspoon sesame oil
- 1 teaspoon minced garlic - Cooked brown rice for serving

- Instructions:

1. In a skillet, heat sesame oil over medium-high heat.
2. Add minced garlic and mixed vegetables to the skillet. Stir-fry for 3-4 minutes until vegetables are tender- crisp.
3. Add cooked lentils to the skillet and stir-fry for an additional 2 minutes.
4. Pour soy sauce and hoisin sauce over the lentil and vegetable mixture, tossing to combine.
5. Serve over cooked brown rice.

39. Baked Salmon with Lemon-Dill Sauce

- Ingredients:

- 2 salmon fillets
- Juice and zest of 1 lemon
- 1 teaspoon dried dill
- Salt and pepper to taste - 2 tablespoons Greek yogurt

- Instructions:

1. Preheat the oven temperature to 375°F (190 °C).

2. On a baking sheet lined with parchment paper, Place salmon fillets.

3. Sprinkle lemon zest, dried dill, salt, and pepper over the salmon.

4. Bake in the preheated oven for 12-15 minutes, or until the salmon flakes easily with a fork.

5. In a small bowl, mix Greek yogurt with lemon juice.

6. Drizzle the lemon-dill sauce over the baked salmon before serving.

Conclusion:

As we wrap up our journey through "Elder Women's Diabetic Delights: Flavorful Recipes for Blood Sugar Management," it's clear that this isn't just a cookbook – it's your partner in crafting a healthier, tastier life. Throughout these pages, we've explored the magic that happens when nourishing food and great flavor come together, all while keeping your blood sugar in check.

We've been right there with you, understanding the unique challenges that come with age and diabetes. By embracing these challenges, we've uncovered a treasure trove of simple yet effective ways to make your daily meals a celebration of well-being.

But let's talk about those recipes – oh, the flavors! We've taken your favorites and given them a wholesome twist, proving that eating smart doesn't mean sacrificing on taste. From that zesty Lemon-Garlic Shrimp to the heartwarming Lentil and Vegetable Soup, these recipes aren't just about eating; they're about savoring life.

Beyond the kitchen, we've dived into the art of staying active, finding your calm, and navigating the real world while keeping your health on track. These aren't just strategies; they're the tools to paint a canvas of vibrant living.

As you close this book, remember this isn't the end; it's a fresh beginning. A new chapter where you're the chef, the artist, the architect of your well-being. These recipes aren't just instructions; they're your passport to a life filled with energy, joy, and a sprinkle of culinary magic.

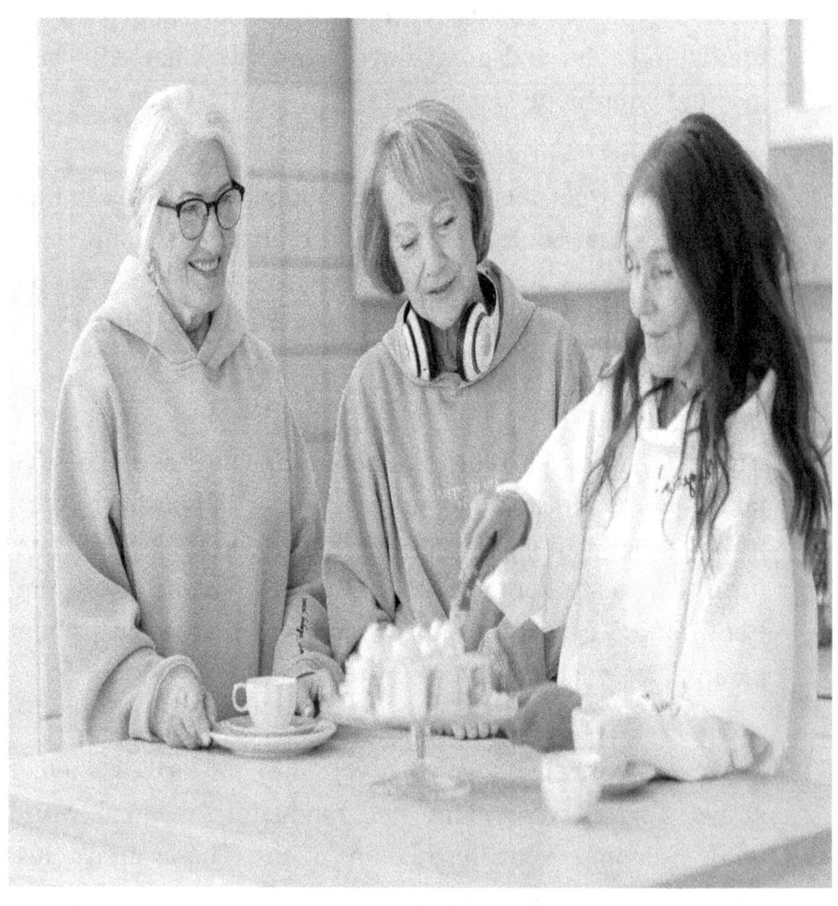

Thanks for Reading:

Dear Friend,

Before we part ways, we want to express our heartfelt gratitude for joining us on this flavorful journey through "Elder Women's Diabetic Delights." Your dedication to your well-being and your zest for savoring life are truly inspiring.

We hope this book has been more than just words on paper. We hope it's become a trusted companion in your kitchen, guiding you towards meals that dance on your taste buds while keeping your blood sugar in check. Your commitment to nurturing your health is something to be celebrated.

As you embark on your culinary adventures, remember that each recipe is a step towards a healthier, happier you. The kitchen is your canvas, and the ingredients are your paint. With every stir, sprinkle, and sizzle, you're creating a masterpiece of well-being.

Thank you for being a part of this journey. Here's to a future filled with delicious discoveries, vibrant health, and many more heart-warming meals.

With a plateful of gratitude,
Dr Marcia Moss